Belly Diet

The Zero Belly Diet Step-By-Step Guide Which Helps You To Lose Your Belly And Enjoy Your Flat Belly

LELA GIBSON

CONTENTS

Introduction

I want to thank you and congratulate you for buying the book, *"Belly Diet: the Zero Belly Diet Step-By-Step Guide Which Helps You to Lose Your Belly and Enjoy Your Flat Belly"*.

This book has lots of actionable information on how to lose your belly fat.

Do you desire a flat tummy? If you do, meet the zero belly diet that trims your tubby tummy and whittles your waist into shape. A flat tummy is a dream for most. You may be a middle-aged person who is not sure how, what, or when it happened, your body just turned into a fat 'packing machine' and before you knew it, there the pot belly was. Perhaps you allowed yourself the luxury of heavy drinking or binge eating and you could now use some help to get rid of that belly fat. If you have belly fat, even when you are not overweight, you can take certain steps to get rid of that fat.

This book gives you the most advanced, tried and proven strategy that will strip away that fat, rev up your metabolism, balance your digestive health, minimize/completely eliminate bloating, and help you have strong and lean abdominal muscles without wasting endless hours at the gym or almost starving yourself.

While there is no shortage of diets that can help you lose belly fat, none is as efficient and quick as the zero belly diet. This diet targets the abdominal fat and deactivates the fatty cells along the abdominal cavity, which in this case are the visceral fatty tissues that usually accumulate in your tummy. These fatty tissues are hazardous because they increase inflammation and may increase the chances of developing some health complications such as cancer, diabetes, arthritis, heart disease, brain degenerative diseases and many others. It does not stop there.

Unhealthy accumulation of visceral fatty tissues can also wear away your muscle tissues, fiddle with your hormone levels, bring down your sex drive, and possibly drive you into depression. Fortunately, you do not have to let it get to that point: you can use the zero belly diet to get rid of accumulated belly fat, and thanks to this book, you will have all you need to get started with the belly diet.

Thanks again for buying this book, I hope you enjoy it!

To help you understand just how revolutionary the zero belly diet is, let's start by understanding the science behind the zero belly diet.

The Science Behind The Zero Belly Diet

To gain weight, you have to eat more calories than your body needs. On the other hand, to lose weight, your body should burn more calories than you eat. While this is the case, have you ever wondered how some people comfortably weigh around 135 pounds (61 kg) without having to adopt a diet, limit their calorie intake, or become gym rats?

Have you also ever wondered how other people weigh in excess of 240 pounds (109 kg) and struggle to shed even a small margin of that weight even though they work out frequently? Why do some children seem to inherit the fat genes from their parents? Does this mean weight gain or subsequent loss is genetic and some of us are fat or lean because our ancestors were so? These questions are ones that have been lingering in the minds of many dieticians and nutritionists for many decades.

The answer is that weight gain is NOT genetic based: its basis is **epigenetics,** which is study of potentially heritable changes in gene expression (inactive against active genes), which does not entail changes in the underlying DNA sequence. In simple terms, it is how biological mechanisms such as age or lifestyle and environmental factors such as stress, chemical exposure, and **diet** switch genes on and off.

A study published in the Journal Advance Nutrition in 2014 revealed that diabetic and obese persons have epigenetic markers that contain different patterns to persons who are not diabetic or obese. In simple terms, this is evidence that there is an alteration of fat genes of obese people.

David Zinczenko, an expert in the field of Nutritional Genomics, which is the study of how various foods interact with particular genes, spent a large part of his career studying belly fat, how it comes to be, and its effects on human beings. He discovered that some of the foods you eat end up turning on your 'fat genes'.

After the activation of these fat genes, it causes a supposedly irrevocable weight gain. However, there are other foods—covered in another chapter in this book—that 'short circuit' or switch off these fat genes. Once these parts of your DNA switch off, instead of storing it, your body starts burning fat.

What you eat or do not eat determines which genes turn on or off, and when. Mr. Zinczenko believes counting the calories you consume is not an efficient pathway to permanent weight loss nor is it sustainable. On the other hand, eating the right way alters everything. This brings us to the belly diet and the foods you should eat and avoid. Let us learn more about this in the next chapter.

Belly Diet: Foods To Eat

To burn fat, which as you now know, means you have to deactivate the 'store fat' genes, you should eat the following foods that activate fat burning in the body:

Protein

5 ounces of Poultry (lean chicken or turkey): Make sure the poultry you eat is skinless or lean (no less than 93% lean meats). Poultry meat is three times more effective at fighting belly fat. It is high in Vitamin B12, DHA omega 3 acids, and methonine.

These three nutrients are critically important in weight loss since they play a key role in turning off the genes linked with insulin resistance and obesity. This halts fat cells from accumulating in the belly.

As you start integrating poultry into your diet, ensure you only eat white poultry meat. The darker one has excessive fat content.

5 ounces of lean red meat (consume this once or twice): As you purchase the meat, make sure it is no less than 90% lean. The most preferred cut is a sirloin cut from a grass fed animal. Lean red meat is rich in vitamin B12, a nutrient known for fueling the fight against weight gain by improving the body's sensitivity to insulin.

5 ounces of fish: Go for wild caught fish and avoid farmed fish because the latter has different kinds of toxins that are harmful to your health. Tuna is a readily available and affordable type of fish whose benefits are immense. Not only is it a good source of protein, it is also rich in **omega-3 docosahexaenoic acid (DHA)**. This fatty acid has the unique ability of turning off the belly fat genes.

As for salmon, a study published in the International Journal of Obesity discovered that while on a low calorie diet, eating three 5-ounce servings of salmon every week leads to a loss of roughly 2.2 pounds each week.

Methionine is another nutrient found in some fishes. The role of Methionine is to reverse the genes responsible for obesity and insulin resistance. Rich sources of methionine are halibut, cold-water fish, freshwater fish (pike and sunfish), poultry, lean meats, and eggs.

5 ounces of eggs: In addition to being rich protein sources, eggs are rich in choline, a fat burning nutrient. Researchers believe choline turns off the genes that cause visceral fat accumulation. Eggs are the leading source of choline but you can also derive choline from lean meats, poultry, collard greens, and seafood.

Legumes: This category includes all kinds of beans, peas, and lentils. These foods all have a nutrient called **genistein.** This compound is very helpful when it comes to switching off the fat genes that cause obesity and belly fat accumulation. It also reduces the body's ability to store fat. Genistein is also present in peanuts and peanut butter.

A study found that people who ate four servings of legumes each week lost a significant amount of weight and their LDL cholesterols reduced as compared to people on a diet without legumes.

High protein plants: Some plants contain a very important type of amino acid called betaine. Examples of such high protein plants are oats, quinoa and brown rice, green tea, leafy greens, and brightly colored vegetables (such as beetroot and spinach).

Betaine is a plant based amino acid that works on a genetic level to switch off the genes responsible for accumulation of fatty cells in the visceral area as well as those that increase the risk of diabetes, liver steatosis (fatty liver), and insulin resistance.

Fiber

2 to 3 heaped cups of leafy green vegetables and non-starchy vegetables: Leafy green vegetables have a nutrient called **sulforaphane**. This compound acts directly on the genes that determine 'adipocyte differentiation'. In other words, sulforaphane shuts down the genes responsible for turning stem cells into fat cells.

When your body has a sufficient amount of this nutrient, it halts weight gain and you begin to lose belly fat, even when you eat tons of calories. This compound is in kales, arugula, collard greens, and watercress. You can also find Sulforaphane in horseradish spices.

Leafy greens also have a type of water-soluble vitamin B called **folate** or **vitamin B9**. This compound turns off genes for adiposity, belly fat, and insulin resistance. Folate is also present in green tea, seafood, grains, nuts and legumes, liver, edible yeast, dairy products, and brightly colored vegetables (asparagus, Brussels Sprouts, lettuce, tomatoes, and spinach).

Fresh Fruits (eat two servings every day): Anthocyanin is the substance that gives red fruits that reddish hue. The function of this substance is to deactivate the genes responsible for fat accumulation. Whenever you pay your grocery store a visit, get into the habit of picking up red fruits over green ones. For example, you can pick up grapes, apples, watermelons, pomegranates, cherries, and red-fleshed peaches. Red cabbage is also a rich source of anthocyanin.

In some other cases, this pigment gives other fruits a dark purple or blue hue rather than red. For example, this pigment is what gives eggplants, plums, black currant, blueberries, blackberries, raspberries, cranberries, and elderberries their dark purple or blue hue. Other surprise fruits such as bananas are also rich in this substance especially considering that they are usually yellow.

On another note, substances called **phenolic compounds** are in red-bellied stone fruits such as plums and peaches. These nutrients are an essential part of the human diet because of their antioxidant properties. More importantly, they also shut down the fat genes that cause obesity and belly fat.

½ a cup of cooked grains: Grains are a great source of insoluble fibers that reduce blood cholesterol. Your gut houses over 80 million healthy bacteria. The insoluble fibers feed these healthy bacteria to help them fight against inflammation and fat gain. This happens when your gut produces **butyrate,** a fatty acid whose function is to reduce inflammation caused by body fat.

When you make grains that have insoluble fiber part of your diet, the body produces a hormone called **ghrelin** whose function is to control hunger, which keeps you from overeating. Types of grain high in fiber include buckwheat, barley, kamut, millet, wheat bran, oats, and quinoa

Amaranth is high in fiber and choke full of monounsaturated fats that lessen body inflammation. This grain also has magnesium that reduces your appetite.

Another important type of grain is Teff. Compared to other types of grain, Teff has unusual high protein content. Moreover, it has 4 times the amount of calcium and twice as much iron as quinoa. Calcium and iron are nutrients associated with lowered body weight and a reduction or a complete halt of weight gain.

Fats and Oils

You still need to consume dietary fats and oils so that your body can lose weight and function appropriately. Some people believe consuming fats and oils leads to weight gain. This is not true. In fact, you should eat healthy fats because healthy fats increase your metabolism, suppress hunger levels, and speed up nutrient absorption all around the body. To achieve this, you must avoid all sorts of unhealthy fats. For example, you should avoid the Trans fats in margarines and lard.

Listed below is a comprehensive list of some of the healthy fats you should include in your diet and the role they play in ensuring you strip away the fat around your abdomen:

Avocado oil

Avocado oil is rich in heart healthy monounsaturated fats that contain your hunger and decrease cholesterol levels in your body. It also has potassium; potassium banishes bloating. Avocado oil also has vitamin E and B. The constituents of this nutrient rich oil is what makes it a 'must have' in many other diets including the 'paleo diet'.

Avocado oil has a lovely mild avocado scent and a light nutty taste that makes it superiorly suited for use as a salad dressing. You can also drizzle it on a fishmeal, bread, or home baked pizza. Avocado oil is also ideal for use in fruit salads especially those that contain watermelons, oranges, or grapefruit.

Walnut oil

Walnut oil has a rich nutty and roasted flavor. A diet consisting of walnuts and walnut oil helps keep diastolic blood pressure down and can equip your body with a better stress mechanism response. Walnut oil has more omega-3 fatty acid than any other type of nut oil. It is also rich in polyunsaturated fatty acids that increase the rate of calorie break down triggered by the zero belly diet.

Walnut oil makes a perfect salad dressing especially when mixed with olive oil, a pinch of salt, ground cumin powder, sherry vinegar, and a sprinkle of pepper. Do not cook or bake with walnut oil: it does not do well under extreme temperatures.

Coconut oil

Coconut oil is popular oil derived from the flesh of fresh coconuts. Its magic ingredient is Lauric acid. Lauric acid is a medium chain saturated fatty acid that has the ability to convert very easily into energy once in the body, something that does not happen with other fatty acids.

According to a research study published in the American Journal of Clinical Nutrition, Coconut oil also has three more fatty acids namely **caprylic acid**, **capric acid**, and **caproic acid** that all increase fat metabolism, which means they turn your body into a fat burning machine while helping you manage food cravings.

Coconut oil is one of the few oils that reduce the levels of cholesterol in your body while at the same time improving your food. A study conducted at the Federal University of Alagoas in Brazil discovered that coconut oil plays a major role in weight loss while improving levels of cholesterol in the body.

Coconut oil can be a great substitute for butter. For example, you can use it to bake cookies or cakes, or use it to fry some foods. Coconut oil also features prominently in Zero Belly Diet Smoothies to create a new and delicious twist in your smoothies.

When mixed with salt, garlic powder, and pepper and then sprinkled over homemade baked sweet potato fries or toast, it adds an exciting flavor. Because it breaks down, which renders useless its active fatty acids, you should be careful not to use coconut oil in cooking that requires the use of extreme heat such as deep-frying.

Olive Oil

Extra virgin olive oil increases the levels of serotonin in the blood; serotonin is a hormone associated with satiety. It can also help you control hunger even for as long as up to four hours. Olive oil also has an antioxidant called polyphenol that fights off diseases such as cancer, brain degeneration, and osteoporosis.

You can use extra virgin olive oil as a salad dressing. You can also use it to cook some dishes especially vegetables. For cooking purposes however, you can use regular or light olive oil.

Canola Oil

Extracted from the seeds of the canola plant in the broccoli family, canola oil is popular as a rich source of a type of omega-3 acid called **alpha-linolenic acid (ALA)**, something research has shown to play a pivotal role in weight maintenance. Moreover, this oil has a near perfect 2½: 1 ratio of omega-6 to omega-3 fatty acids. Persons with a dietary ratio similar to this can effectively battle cancer, asthma, or arthritis.

The benefit of canola oil is that it can endure extreme heat conditions. This makes it a good option for cooking your dishes. If you are super sensitive to strong aromas, canola oil is fairly neutral and does not dominate a dish.

Peanut Oil

Peanut oil is burgeoning with **oleic acid,** a type of monounsaturated fatty acid that reduces appetite while encouraging weight loss. Research has also shown that oleic acid boosts memory. Like canola oil, peanut oil has a high smoke point and you can therefore use it for frying and other forms of dish preparation that involve extreme heating such as pan searing and wok cooking.

Spices

For spices opt for:

Black pepper

For ages, this spice has found use as medication for treating abdomen troubles and inflammation. Research has also discovered that black pepper contains a compound called **piperine.** Piperine reacts in the body to cause adipogenesis, which is interference with the production of new fat cells. The result of this process is the reduction of body fat, reduction in waist size, and a drastic plummet of cholesterol levels. You can sprinkle some black pepper on your salads or grilled meat.

Cayenne

A research study published in the American Journal of Clinical Nutrition discovered that consumption of capsaicin (a substance found in cayenne that produces a hot sensation) helps burn visceral fatty tissues.

Another study conducted by Canadian scientists showed that people who ate appetizers containing this substance reduced their calorie intake by an average of 200 calories in their meals than those who did not. Capsaicin is also present in hot sauces. You can use Cayenne to season grilled meat, fish, or eggs.

Mustard Seeds

Researchers at the Oxford Polytechnic Institute discovered that when you add 1 teaspoon of prepared mustard to your meal–equivalent to roughly 5 calories; it boosts your metabolism rate by 25 percent, a boost that lasts hours after your meal.

In another study published in the Asian Journal of Clinical Nutrition, researchers discovered that the abdominal fatty tissues of rats reduced after the rats fed on lard supplemented with mustard oil. The substance that caused this reduction is allyl isothiocyanates, the substance that gives mustard its unique flavor.

Cinnamon

Cinnamon contains **polyphenols;** polyphenols are antioxidants that increase insulin sensitivity. One research study published in the Archives of Biochemistry and Biophysics revealed that consumption of cinnamon decreases the accumulation of visceral fatty tissues. The American Journal of Clinical Nutrition has a series of publications about research studies that show that adding a heaped teaspoonful of cinnamon on starchy food helps keep insulin spikes at bay and stabilizes blood sugar levels.

You can sprinkle cinnamon on smoothies or oats for breakfast. You can also use it as an ingredient in cookies, cakes, pies, or pudding to give your meal an aromatic and a sweet, savory flavor.

Zero Belly Diet Drinks

Drinks make up an integral part of belly diet foods. Below are some tasty drinks:

Smoothies

These smoothies are all plant based protein drinks that have the power to bring dramatic changes to your body. To make the simple yet powerful drinks that will trim your tummy and excessive body fats, you only need a blender, and the ingredients discussed in this section of this guide.

Banana Split

This smoothie has two main ingredients namely 70% dark chocolate (cacao) and a banana. This duo has the ability to accelerate the production of a colonic substance called **butyrate** whose function is to shut down the genes responsible for fat storage.

To make this, simply blend all the following ingredients, add two ice cubes, and top with a cherry:

2 dark chocolate squares

1 frozen banana

1 teaspoonful of vanilla extract

1 scoop of vanilla plant-based protein powder

4 pitted cherries and 1 more for the topping

½ cup of unsweetened almond milk

2 ice cubes

Ginger Smoothie

Ginger is a health booster thanks to the amount of phytonutrients it has. It is advisable to use fresh ginger instead of powdered ginger since the latter is not as potent. To keep ginger fresher for longer, dice it and freeze it so that whenever you need to use it, you can simply defrost and then grate it. Simply blend all the following ingredients:

1 tablespoon of fresh, peeled and chopped ginger

1 cup of unsweetened almond milk

1 teaspoon of ground flaxseed

1 scoop of plain plant-based protein powder

¼ cup of frozen banana

½ cup of frozen strawberries

A dash of ground pepper

Water to blend (optional)

Apple Smoothie

According to a study at the University of Western Australia, the **Pink Lady** variety of apples is one on the richest in nutrients. You should therefore pick these in abundance the next time you shop for apples. This smoothie is majorly an autumnal fruit blend of apples, cinnamon, and vanilla that will leave you licking your lips in delight. It consists of:

½ unpeeled Pink Lady apple, quartered and seeded

¼ frozen banana

1 teaspoon of flaxseed oil

1 scoop of plain plant-based protein powder

3 dashes of ground cinnamon

Water to blend

Strawberry Pistachio Smoothie

The pistachio is a member of the cashew family long cherished as the symbol of robust health and wellness since time immemorial. Pistachios are an excellent source of monounsaturated fatty acids and **oleic acid** that help suppress cravings while encouraging weight loss.

Further, the oleic acid in pistachios increases the amount of good cholesterol known as High Density Lipoprotein (HDL) and decreases the amount of bad cholesterol known as Low Density Lipoprotein (LDL) in the body. To make this awesome fruity smoothie, mix:

¼ cup of pistachios

½ cup of frozen strawberries

½ avocado, peeled, pitted, and cubed

1 teaspoonful of vanilla extract

1 scoop of vanilla protein powder

3 ice cubes

Water to blend (necessary)

Peach Oat Smoothie

Peaches have a sweet flesh, a soft skin, and they are the staple fruits of the summer. A standard peach that is around 2¾ inches in diameter has 68 calories. This is the reason why it is ideal for weight control. Moreover, peaches are naturally sweet and if you have a sweet tooth, you can substitute harmful artificial sugars for healthy peaches since sugar is one of the major causes of weight gain.

½ peach

½ frozen banana

1 teaspoon of ground flaxseed

2 tablespoons of rolled oats

1 scoop of vanilla plant-based protein powder

½ cup of unsweetened almond milk

Water to blend (optional)

Peachy Banana

The main ingredients in this drink are peaches and bananas, polar opposites. Peaches are storehouses of antioxidants but offer very little calories. On the other hand, bananas are high in fiber and calories. To make this smoothie:

½ banana

1 cup of frozen peaches

1 teaspoon of vanilla extract

1 scoop of vanilla plant-based protein powder

1 cup of unsweetened almond milk

½ cup of ice cubes

Water to blend (optional)

Green Smoothies

Parsley Strawberry Smoothie

Parsley is an underappreciated food. You may have been thinking that parsley is nothing if not a decorative garnish that accompanies restaurant meals. However, parsley is packed with nutrients and when you combine it with other healthy super foods such as chia and watercress, you will reap unique health benefits.

Simply blend all the following ingredients:

¼ cup of fresh parsley (leaves and stems alike)

½ cup of watercress

½ cup of frozen banana

½ cup of frozen strawberries

1 teaspoon of chia seeds

1 scoop of plain protein powder

Water

Green Hemp Smoothie

The main ingredients in this green smoothie are chia and hemp, a combination that gives you a super dose of omega-3 fatty acids. Hemp seeds are a gift of nature and some claim they are the most nutritious seeds in the world. It is difficult to argue against that statement because they are a complete protein and have the most concentrated balance of vitamins, enzymes, proteins, and essential fats. To make this green smoothie, blend:

1 teaspoon of hemp seeds

½ tablespoon of chia seeds

½ frozen banana

½ cup of unsweetened almond milk

¾ cup of baby kale

1 scoop of vanilla protein powder

Water to blend

Apple Romaine Smoothie

Also known as cos, romaine is a variety of lettuce that not only excites your taste buds, but is also rich in nutrients. This impressive leafy green lettuce has more fiber than any other lettuce variety; it also has a lot of water. To make, blend the following:

1 cup of romaine lettuce

½ cup of spinach

½ cup of unsweetened almond milk

½ unpeeled apple, seeded and quartered

1 scoop of protein powder

1 tablespoon of chia seeds

Water

Green Tea Smoothie

This recipe allows you to combine tea with a smoothie. The green tea in this case functions as a smoothie enhancer:

1 cup of green tea

½ frozen banana

1 scoop of vanilla protein powder

1/8 of an avocado

2 tablespoons of fresh lemon juice

Water to blend

Chocolate and Nutty Smoothies

Chocolate Bean Smoothie

For a thick smoothie rich in protein and fiber, use black beans (canned or precooked).

¼ cup of black beans

½ frozen banana

1 teaspoon of nutmeg

¼ cup of chocolate protein powder

1 cup of unsweetened almond milk

Water to blend

Steel Abs Smoothie

For this smoothie recipe, use almond butter made from dry-roasted almonds with a bit of palm fruit oil to give the butter that creamy feel:

2 teaspoons of almond butter

¾ cup of unsweetened almond milk

¾ frozen banana

1 scoop of chocolate or vanilla protein powder

Water to blend

Savory Smoothies

Sweet Potato Smoothie

The main ingredients here are sweet potatoes and bananas, both of which are starchy foods. That is why there is an extra punch of cinnamon in there to ensure stabilization of your blood sugar and prevent insulin spikes:

½ skinned, cooked and cooled sweet potato

½ frozen banana

1 cup of unsweetened almond milk

½ teaspoon of cinnamon

1 scoop of plain plant-based protein powder

Water to blend (optional)

Zero Belly Diet Teas And Other Drinks

The following are great teas and drinks for weight loss:

Green Tea

Green tea has a form of catechin called **Epigallocatechin-3-gallate (EGCG), a** catechin shown to blast adipose tissues by accelerating the rate of metabolism. An increased rate of metabolism triggers the freeing of fat from fatty tissues and increases the liver's efficiency to burn. This compound also stabilizes blood sugar levels.

White Tea

White tea works in many ways to improve fat burning. First, it disrupts the creation of new fat cells while boosting lipolysis (the process of breaking down stored fat). White tea is rich in **catechins**. Catechins are antioxidants that set off the release of fatty cells. These compounds also accelerate the liver's ability to convert fat into energy.

Rooibos Tea

This tea is naturally red, sweet, and made from the leaves of the Rooibos herb. Some South African scientists studied this herb and found it contains **polyphenols** and **flavonoids,** both of which inhibit the process of adipogenesis by as far as 22%. As stated earlier, adipogenesis is the development of new fat cells. Moreover, these compounds play a part in fat metabolism.

Matcha

Matcha is a Japanese tea made from the leaves of the tencha plant. Matcha is a Japanese word that literally translated means 'powdered tea.' This means the leaves are stone ground to form a bright green fine powder that is then used to prepare tea.

The concentration of **epigallocatechin-3-gallate** in this incredible tea is a whopping 137 times higher than the quantity found in most green teas. A single serving of this tea offers 4 grams of protein, which is more protein than what you will find in one egg white. You can make the powder yourself and use it for preparing tea. You can also use it in smoothies, lattes, milkshakes, and iced drinks.

Red Wine

Have a glass or two every week: research shows that this helps the body burn fat. According to a 2015 study published in the Nutritional Biochemistry, red wine is the best possible source of a micronutrient called **resveratrol**.

Resveratrol effectively shuts down the genes that cause belly fat, obesity, and liver steatosis (abnormal accumulation of fat around the liver). Resveratrol is principally present in the skin of grapes. The alcohol in the wine extracts the resveratrol out of the skin to form a percentage that is higher than what you normally find in grape juice. If you leave some wine to sit on a glass overnight, you will find flaky and reddish-purple sediment at the bottom. That is resveratrol.

Zero Belly Snacks

You read the title right: several snacks help you burn belly fat. Losing that stubborn belly fat does not mean that you have to take yourself through a boot camp like ordeal: there still is room for fun in your meals. It is possible to snack and lose belly fat; you just have to do it smartly and know what to eat.

Here are some snacks that will help your body burn fat:

Shrimp Stack

You perhaps don't consider shellfish as a 'grab and go' snack food. However, you can put this treat together in just a few minutes. This is especially so if you have pre-cooked your shrimp beforehand.

If you combine this with some Greek yogurt and half an avocado, it is a protein powerhouse. It will give you 10 grams of protein per serving and an additional 5 grams of fiber. All of this will be in a 129-calorie package, which is impressive in its own right.

Try this simple shrimp stack recipe:

Calories: 129

Ingredients

½ teaspoon of fresh lime juice

1 tablespoon of fat-free plain Greek yogurt

¼ avocado, chopped

¼ teaspoon of jalapeno sauce

1 crisp rye flatbread

Chopped fresh parsley and cracked black pepper (this is for garnish)

5 cooked large shrimp

Preparation

Stir the yogurt, sauce, lime juice, and avocado and spread on cracker. Top with parsley, shrimp, and pepper.

A few things to know:

Shrimp stack offers a wholesome package of bulk, flavor, and taste. It is ideal when you are looking to have a filling snack. It will only take 10 minutes to have shrimp stack ready. The ingredients laid out are sufficient for one serving.

Shrimp is low in fat and calories (hence the impressively low 129 calorie amount) but comes packed with protein. Each of your servings will consist of 5 shrimp, fat free Greek yogurt, heart-healthy avocado, some jalapeno, spices and lime juice placed on rye flatbread.

Skim Milk And An Apple

Just about any fruit will make a good snack. However, you will want to pair it with some protein to make it a little more satisfying. You may be wondering, "Why not pair it with carbohydrates?" Well, the body uses carbohydrates relatively quickly, which means after eating carbs, you are likely to feel hungry soon after, which will make you want to snack again.

Moreover, consuming too many calories will do you no favors in your attempts to lose belly fat. Protein such as skim milk will help sustain your hunger and energy levels for at least a couple of hours.

Take one large apple and one cup of skim milk. This combination will give you 5 grams of fiber and 10 grams of protein for just over 200 calories.

Sunflower Lentil Spread With Pita Bread

Lentils are excellent sources of iron. What does iron have to do with shedding belly fat? Iron is a nutrient known to boost metabolism when ingested. Statistics have shown that about 20% of all Americans do not get enough iron in their day-to-day lives.

The recipe provided here will make 4, 180 calorie servings. You will have 10 grams of fiber and 10 grams of protein per serving, and it will keep you full until your next meal arrives.

Try this sunflower lentil spread recipe:

Calories: 180

Ingredients:

1 15-ounce can of lentils, rinsed and then drained

¼ teaspoon of salt

1 tablespoon of lemon juice

¼ teaspoon of pepper

2 tablespoons of sunflower seeds

1 scallion, finely diced

1 celery stalk, finely diced

2 halved pitas

2 tablespoons of chopped fresh parsley

Preparation:

Combine the lemon juice, lentils, salt, and pepper in a blender and process until smooth

Stir in the sunflower seeds, scallions, celery, and parsley

Microwave the pita at HIGH one minute.

Serve with spread.

A few things to know:

Lentils will give you a solid amount of resistance starch. Resistance starch is a requisite in your daily diet, and you require at least 10 grams of it in a day. This snack will give you at least one third of this while also helping you cut out that stubborn belly fat.

Cottage Cheese-Filled Avocado

This is yet another fruit and protein/dairy combo. You will snack on this one when you are craving something 'rich', savory, and with a creamy feel to it.

Remove the pit from one half of your avocado and fill the space with about 2 ounces of 1% cottage cheese. For just over 200 calories, you will get 7 grams of fiber and 9 grams of protein. The icing on the cake is that you do not have to deal with any dirty dishes!

Canned Tuna On Whole Wheat Crackers

If you are not fond of dairy and would like to avoid it whenever you can, a can of tuna, packaged in water, is a great source of lean protein. It also comes with a healthy dose of Omega-3s. For about 200 calories, you will have 3 ounces of tuna and six whole-wheat crackers. This will give you 20 grams of protein and 3 grams of fiber.

Special Mention: Nuts And Seeds

Eating almonds will help you lose weight in that midsection. According to a study published in the Journal of the American Heart Association sometime in 2015, almonds help drastically reduce belly fat when used as a substitute for other snacks. The researchers split a group of 48 test subjects into two groups. They had one group snack on 1.5 ounces of almonds every day while they had the other group snack on muffins with the same calories. After only two weeks, the almond group lost more fat than the muffin. You can as well take macadamia nuts; they are just as great as almonds.

Some other snacks that you can take to supercharge the rate at which you see the belly fat coming off include the following:

- Fries made with sweet potatoes, pepper, sea salt and coconut oil (all you need to do is to bake them) can supercharge your metabolism, fight insulin resistance and ultimately help in losing belly fat.

- Creamy deviled eggs made combining hardboiled eggs with smoked paprika, mustard, relish and homemade mayonnaise.

- Roasted pumpkin seeds: all you need to do is to toss the pumpkin seeds inside some pepper, salt and olive oil then bake for a few minutes.

- Avocado-tomato salad, which you make using a few sliced tomatoes, avocado and balsamic vinegar

- Strawberries mixed with balsamic vinegar

- Eggs baked in avocado

- Watermelon mixed with lime juice, salted pistachios and cayenne pepper

Tip: Feel free to add natural peanut butter to any of your recipes; it is a great addition if you want to supercharge your metabolism.

Belly Diet Workout Program

Yes, your diet is important. The foods you eat have a direct impact on the amount of fat your body stores. If you eat, more calories than you use up, you will definitely end up gaining weight and storing belly fat. This is why it is important to create a caloric deficit in order to lose belly fat. A good workout program should help you to lose the belly fat. Some great exercises include:

Move about

You need to keep moving throughout the day so that you can use up calories. The more you move, the more you burn fat and this includes belly fat. Don't sit down for more than one hour before moving. Stand up and take a walk around your house. Lift something up to get your heart pumping. Do some chores and walk the dog. In other words, find various opportunities to burn fat.

Walk

Walking is a great way to burn belly fat. However, you need to get the most out of it. This means walking for 45 minutes to 1 hour at least 3 times a week. Therefore, map out your route and find comfortable walking shoes. Determine what time you will be walking and stick to it. If you cannot walk for that long, start with a 5-minute walk and then increase the duration over time. The great thing about walking is that walking exercises various muscles in your body including your stomach muscles.

You can train yourself to walk more throughout the day. For example, you can take the stairs more and you can walk to some places instead of taking the bus. You can even alight a stop earlier and walk the rest of the way.

Simple exercises

In addition to walking, you also need to engage in some exercises. You don't need to get a gym membership in order to do this. You can do some exercises right in your home or even at work. These include:

Chair squats

- Find a sturdy chair and stand in front of it with your feet about shoulder width apart. One leg should be at one o'clock and the other at eleven o'clock.

- Keep your chest area straight as you lower yourself into a squat position. Your upper legs should just touch your chair.

- Drive up and push your knees outwards so that they don't collapse inwards. Dig your heels into the floor as you do this.

- As you reach the top, make sure you squeeze your thighs and flutes.

- Repeat the exercise 15-20 times.

As you become more comfortable with the exercise, you can remove the chair and take a moment to pause at the bottom of each rep.

Chair dips

- Find a sturdy chair and sit on the edge. Your hands should grip it at the edge on both sides and your legs should be straightened just in front of you.

- Once you're in position, start lowering your bum towards the floor while flexing at your elbows. Go as low as you can.

- Go back to the starting position and make sure you squeeze your triceps as you do.

- Repeat the exercise 15-20 times.

If the exercise feels a bit difficult, you can bend your legs and bring your feet a bit closer to your body.

Split squat/lunges

- Stand in a lunge position by placing your right foot in front of your left foot.

- Slowly proceed to move your left foot (back foot) towards the floor. The front knee should bend simultaneously as you move your left foot. Keep your chest straight and facing forward.

- Go back to the starting position; you should drive up through the front leg. Squeeze both your thighs and your glutes as you reach the top.

- Repeat the exercise 15 times per leg

Narrow grip dress press

- In a press up position, form a diamond shape by placing your thumbs and index fingers close together.

- Proceed to bend both your elbows and then lower your chest area down towards the ground. You should get as low to the ground as you can without touching it. Once you do, push yourself back to the starting position in a powerful move.

- Remember to keep your flutes and abs tight as you do the exercise. Repeat 15 times.

It would be good to remember that not everyone has the same level of fitness. Ideally, you should aim for 15-20 minutes of exercise. However, you may find it challenging to do more than a few reps of each exercise. Don't be discouraged. Start with the few reps and increase them as you go.

As always, keep in mind that what you are aiming for is caloric deficit. But it wouldn't hurt to firm up your belly muscles even as you lose the belly fat. This will end up better for you in the end. You will lose the fat and look good at the same time.

Losing Belly Fat Tips

In this chapter, we will look at some tips to help you lose belly fat:

Go for brisk walks every morning (before breakfast)

One of the people on the Zero belly diet program, Martha Chesler started taking brisk walks as part of her program and in less than 6 weeks, she had lost 7 inches from her waist. This was possible because it has been proven that exposing yourself to the 8 am and noon sunlight helps reduce your weight gain risks irrespective of your age, calorie intake and activity level. Morning light undercuts your fat genes and synchronizes your metabolism.

In addition, walking before breakfast means that you will be burning calories in a fasted state. This means that instead of burning energy from the food you eat, it will be from your stored fat hence you will lose some belly fat.

Always go for red fruits

Make sure to choose red fruits over the greens ones. For example, choose to eat more watermelons, pink lady or red grapes. This is because red fruits have high levels of flavonoids (the anthocyanins compounds which give the red fruits their color) nutrients which calm the actions of the genes which store fat. In addition, red fruits such as plums help improve the levels of phenolic compounds, which moderate expression of fat genes.

Eat Guacamole

Start including fresh products (like avocados) in your diet and you will be surprised how your weight and belly fat will keep coming off. First, avocados have unsaturated fats that help prevent the storage of belly fat. Secondly, eating fresh and chemical free foods like avocado provides you with monounsaturated fat, which dims your hunger switches hence leading to fat loss. This argument was supported in a study which was published in the Nutrition Journal where they found that people who ate ½ fresh avocado with their lunch meal had a 40% decrease in the desire to eat for some hours afterwards.

Eat peanut butter

Real peanut butter has peanut and some salt as the only ingredients. Peanut butter provides you with tummy filling fiber, metabolism boosting protein and belly slimming monounsaturated fats. In addition, it has genistein compounds, which act directly on obesity genes hence turning them down and reducing your ability to store fat. Beans and lentils have the same hidden weapon (genistein).

Always remember to be careful and look at the ingredients of the peanut butter brand you buy as it may contain some ingredients such as palm oil, sugar or other things, which you can't pronounce, that may undermine all the good things peanut butter is supposed to do.

Drink adequate water

Water is an important part of your diet. This is because many chemical processes taking place in your body require water. In addition, water is effective in flushing out toxins that are known to cause weight gain. Therefore, ensure you take at least 8 glasses of water daily.

Mix up a magic elixir every day

I mentioned earlier that water is very important. However, if you cannot take plain water, you can opt for this magic elixir. Each day, make a large pitcher of spa water (water with slices of whole oranges, grapefruits or lemons) and make an effort of drinking at least 8 glasses before you go to sleep. According to the World Health Organization, citrus fruits have antioxidant delimonene (found in the peel) which stimulates liver enzymes hence helping in flushing toxins from your body and giving sluggish bowels a kick.

Exercise

The New Zealand scientists found that men and women who did 10 minutes exercise before breakfast, lunch and dinner had lowered blood glucose levels (a benefit of fat busting).

Include berries and dark chocolate in your dessert

A study at Louisiana University found that the gut microbes (in the stomach) ferment dark chocolate into heart-healthy anti-inflammatory compounds, which slow down inflammation and insulin resistance genes. The berries you include in your dessert will help speed up the fermentation process hence leading to weight loss and reduced inflammation. Also, another study found that cocoa has antioxidant properties, which can lower your blood sugar levels and prevent you from gaining weight.

Always go for wild salmon

Protein from fish is one of the best ways of boosting your metabolism and fighting fat. However, when it comes to belly fat, always go for the wild fish. This is because you cannot trust farmed fish. Most of the packages will indicate that the farmed fish has 114 mg of belly busting omega 3 fatty acids while in real sense they contain 1900 mg of unhealthy omega 6s.

Always make your own trial mix

A good zero belly diet meal or snack should have fiber, protein and healthy fat. All these nutrients are abundant in a good trial mix but the sad thing is that most of the commercial trial mixes have extra sugar, salt and oils. To be on the safe side, make your own trial mix from your selected nuts, unsweetened dried fruits, pieces of dark chocolate and seeds.

Always include peanuts as they are rich in resveratrol and genistein nutrients, which help slow down the action of your fat-storage genes.

Power up with eggs

Although all your zero belly diet meals have lean, satiating protein, you need a muscle- building macronutrient in your diet, and eggs being one of the easiest and versatile delivery system, you can use it to power up. Also, eggs provide you with choline nutrient (also found in seafood, lean meat and collard green) which attacks your gene mechanism hence triggering your body to store fat around the liver.

Rethink your supplements

If you are used to taking lots of probiotics and vitamins every day, you may want to re- evaluate your diet strategy. A study by ConsumerLam. Com proved that most probiotics do not have as much healthy bacteria as they claim. Well, a daily multivitamin is okay but taking more is not better. In addition, high levels of vitamin B have been associated with diabetes and obesity (because mega-dosing triggers fat genes).

Track your food

Any diet that is geared towards weight loss has to take into account the calories you consume. You cannot lose weight if you eat more calories than you spend. Thus, you need to track the amount of food you eat. Ideally, you should eat between 1600-2000 calories depending on your gender and the amount of physical activity you perform. If you don't move about a lot, you should eat fewer calories.

A good way to track your food is to write on a journal. This will also serve to ensure that you only eat the foods acceptable in the belly diet.

De-stress

It's not unusual to eat a lot when you're stressed. Many people find comfort in food when things are not going right. High carb foods work well to provide that soothing effect to your brain. However, they also contribute to belly fat. It is important to learn how to de-stress for the sake of your health and weight.

Start by identifying the source of stress and determine which ones you can get rid of. Next, determine how to deal with people or situations in your daily life. This will reduce your stress levels. Additionally, you need to spend a bit of time on yourself. Use this time to relax or do something you love. You can perform a physical activity such as walking, dancing, playing basketball or swimming. Such activities will help you relieve stress and they will help you lose belly fat.

I need your help...

We have come to the end of the book. Thank you for reading and congratulations for reading until the end.

I hope this book was able to help you to get an idea about how to lose your belly. Now that you have the belly fat burning formula at your fingertips, you should be confident of achieving exceptional results once you start this diet and as you have seen, this diet is simple and you will still get to enjoy the foods you love.

With the zero belly diet, you can finally change your destiny by overcoming your fat genes to strip away that potbelly and attain a lean body. Most importantly, this diet allows you to take control of your health and life.

To join the zero diet movement and say goodbye to your protruding tummy, forever take action NOW.

Finally, if you enjoyed this book, then I'd like to ask you for a favor, would you be kind enough to leave a review for this book on Amazon? It'd be greatly appreciated!

I want to reach as many people as I can with this book, and more reviews will help me accomplish that!

If you have any questions or problems, please contact us: hello@freedomdestination.com

Thank you and good luck!

Preview Of '20 Easy And Fast Diet Tips For Losing Weight'

Before we start learning about the strategies you can use to lose weight, let's start by highlighting some of the benefits that will come as a result of shedding those extra pounds just to give you extra motivation to want to do something NOW.

Why You Need To Lose Weight

Healthy weight loss has over one hundred benefits; these include emotional and physical benefits. I will dedicate this section to discussing the health benefits that many people (and weight loss/health books) do not pay enough attention to.

1: You Avoid Pre-Diabetes or Type 2 Diabetes

Pre-diabetes/high blood glucose is a condition that develops when the blood sugar levels in your blood move past normal ranges but not enough to qualify as diabetes. When your body stops consistently producing insulin sufficient to meet your body's needs, or the amount produced does not work properly, type 2 diabetes is likely to develop. Being pre-diabetic places you at a very high risk of developing type 2 diabetes.

Being obese or overweight is a proven leading risk factor for type 2 diabetes because carrying excess weight typically makes it hard for cells to respond to insulin, and since the additional fat acts as an insulating layer, it makes it more difficult for the sugar to enter the cells, which results in more circulating blood sugar levels.

Nonetheless, if you are already a pre-diabetic, you can prevent the progression to diabetes by shedding some weight (to reduce the insulating layer on cells so that they respond more to insulin) and trying to maintain a healthy weight.

2: You Keep Your Heart Healthy

When it comes to heart disease, some of the key risk factors are high cholesterol and high blood pressure. Research shows that:

1. Excessive accumulation of body fat makes your body release particular chemicals that occur naturally into the bloodstream, which increases blood pressure, and

2. Being overweight makes the liver produce too much amounts of Low density Lipoprotein (LDL) also called cholesterol. LDL tends to be sticky and gathers in the walls of blood vessels, which causes the narrowing of arteries, a condition called atherosclerosis, which increases your risk of strokes and heart attack.

When you lose weight, your blood pressure often reduces and the liver naturally reduces the amount of LDL it produces.

Royal Adelaide Hospital conducted a research on cardiovascular improvements with respect to a special weight loss program. Their results showed a decrease of cholesterol by 12%, a 10% decrease of LDL, a 5% decrease in diastolic blood pressure, and an 8% decrease in systolic blood pressure.

3: Improved Sleep (and Possible Treatment of Sleep Apnea)

One of the most prominent benefits of losing weight is improved sleep. When you gain excess weight, you gather more soft tissues in the neck; this intensifies the incidence of snoring.

NOTE: Snoring is a result of constricted airways, which obstructs air movement.

Snoring can be a symptom of sleep apnea, a possible life-threatening condition characterized by obstruction of breathing that requires the victim to wake up frequently from sleep to resume breathing.

As a victim of sleep apnea, you rarely remember anything about the episodes of waking many times a night to breathe but even so, this sleep and oxygen deprivation could easily lead to a weak immune system, high blood pressure, heart disease, memory problems, and sexual dysfunction.

When you lose weight, you reduce the amount of fatty tissue in the back of your throat, decrease snoring and the likelihood of the worsening of your health- as aforementioned. You encourage better sleep quality and reduce the risk of developing sleep apnea.

4: Better Joints (Mobile and Pain-Free)

Osteoarthritis (OA) is one of the most common joint disorders. It causes the tissues that protect the joints (cartilage and bone) to wear away. Consequently, the joints become tender and swollen, thus making movement very painful.

When you are overweight, you add to the load placed on the joints that bear the weight such as hips and knees.

NOTE: When you walk, you exert a force of approximately 3-6 times your entire body weight across the knee (read more on this page (check the discussion section) or here), so adding about 10 kg of weight does increase the force on the knees, which is equal to carrying 30-60 kgs^2 extra.

Therefore, a loss of merely 5% of your body weight could reduce the amount of stress placed on the knees, lower back, and hips, and reduce the pain (remember that losing 5kgs is equal to relieving a force of 15-30kgs^2 on the knees). According to doctors, a 10% loss of bodyweight has presented a 28% improvement in knee osteoarthritis symptoms.

5: Improved Fertility

There is epidemiological evidence that proves being obese has negative effects on reproduction. There has not been clarity in the mechanisms underlying the relationship between infertility and obesity but research studies suggest that excess body can lead to a serious offset in the metabolism of sex hormones that produce menstrual disruption and consequently, subfertility.

Moreover, when you are pregnant and overweight, you a more likely to miscarry and (or) develop other medical complications, and in particular, gestational diabetes, pregnancy induced hypertension, thromboembolism, and preeclampsia. There are reports to show that deliveries in obese women show increased rates of labor induction, caesarian section, and problematic labor caused by increased size of the unborn baby.

Additionally, experts report that a baby of an overweight woman is more likely to require more medical attention (admission to neonatal intensive care) and develop congenital defects such as cardiac and neural tube problems.

Moreover, obese individuals are more likely to experience birth related injuries and the likelihood of giving birth to babies with large birth weights, which puts them at risk of birth trauma and a possibility of childhood and probably lifelong obesity. Reducing weight in this case could help you and your baby avoid all these health problems.

Emotional Weight Loss Benefits

The negativity usually around overweight people affects your self-esteem and confidence. Naturally, when you are carrying some excess weight, you will worry about how other people see you and become overly anxious in particular situations. This affects many aspects of your life including your job interactions and performance, school, and your life at home (in the neighborhood).

Losing weight will help you gain confidence and increase your self-worth and self-love; losing weight normally makes you cheerful and as a result, your relationships with other people improve. Most of your fears and anxieties related to being overweight disappear and in general, you live a better life.

Once you regain your confidence, you feel in control. This becomes the status quo once you become comfortable with your new weight. Once you lose the weight, you are more comfortable when making food related decisions.

You also feel and become more honest when you interact with others and can better articulate your thoughts and feelings. You will no longer hold back since you are more self-possessed about your appearance and health.

Now that you know some of the benefits you stand to gain from losing weight, let us discuss the various effortless ways to lose weight.

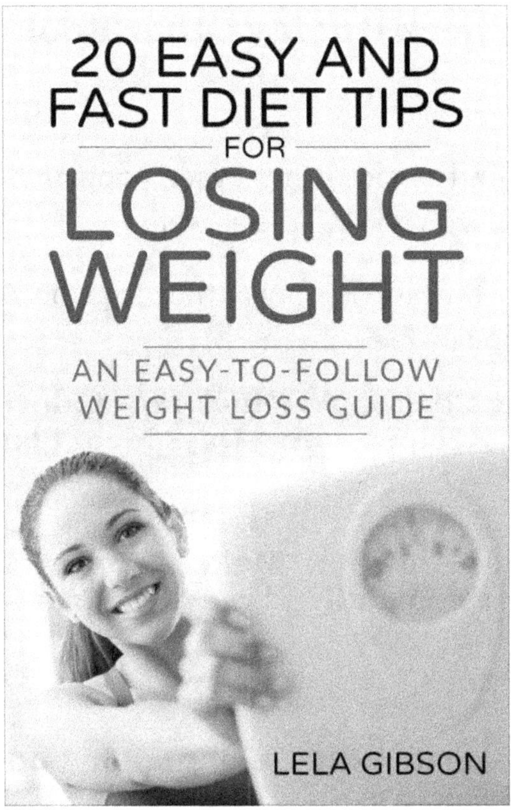

Check out the rest of 20 Easy And Fast Diet Tips For Losing Weight on Amazon, go to: http://amzn.to/2mNtPEg

Check Out My Other Books

Below you'll find some of my other popular books that are popular on Amazon and Kindle as well.

Alternatively, you can visit my author page on Amazon to see other work done by me.

Ketogenic Cookbook: Quick Low Calorie Ketogenic Crockpot Recipes with 7 Days Meal Plan

Freedom: How to Make Money Online and Become Financially Free by Creating Passive Income

Mediterranean Diet: Instant Pot Cookbook with Delicious Recipes

Alice the Superbug

Madison and Astrid's first magical journey

Intermittent Fasting: The Essential Beginners Guide for Women for Weight Loss

Chakra Healing: Chakra Healing and Karmic Awareness for Beginners

SEO 2017 for Growth: The Ultimate Guide to Learn Search Engine Optimization with Internet Marketing Tips

Psychology: How to Analyze People Using Human Psychological Techniques, Body Language Signals, Social Skills and Personality Types

Paleo Smoothies: Recipes to Energize and for Ultimate Health and Weight Loss

Belly Diet Smoothies: Delicious Smoothie Recipes to Flatten Your Belly, Improve Your Gut & Burn Fat

Keto Diet: Keto Diet Guide Cookbook for Beginners with Meal Plan and Simple, Delicious Recipes to Lose Weight and Look Good

Online Business from Scratch: The 9 Step Guide to Building a Profitable and Sustainable Online Business

Weight Loss: 20 Easy And Fast Diet Tips For Losing Weight - An Easy-To-Follow Weight Loss Guide

Ketogenic Cookbook: Ketogenic Cookbook for Beginners with 7 Days Meal Plan

Negative Calorie Diet: Cookbook & Guide Which Will Help You To Burn Body Fat, Lose Weight And Live Healthy

Negative Calorie Diet with Anti-Inflammatory Diet Guide

Make Money Online To Achieve Freedom

Negative Calorie Diet with Smart Fat Guide

Negative Calorie Diet & Clean Eating: Cookbook & Guide Which Will Help You To Burn Body Fat, Lose Weight And Live Healthy

Smart Fat: Cookbook with Fat Meals Which Help You to Lose Weight, Get Healthy and Improve Brain Function

Anti-Inflammatory Diet Guide: The Guide to Reduce Inflammation and Live a Healthy Life Without Pain

Essential Oils: The Young Living Book Guide of Natural Remedies for Beginners for Pets, For Dogs

Clean Eating: Cookbook and Guide to Restore Your Body's Natural Balance and Eat Healthy

Anti-Inflammatory Diet Guide: The Guide to Reduce Inflammation and Live a Healthy Life Without Pain

Dash Diet: Cookbook for Weight Loss with Action Plan and Easy Recipes

Air Fryer Cookbook: Quick, Healthy and Easy Low Carb Air Fryer Recipes

Psychology & Habits Of Highly Effective People Box Set

Leptin Resistance: Leptin Diet to Control Your Hormones, Get Permanent Weight Loss, Cure Obesity and Live Healthy

Negative Calorie Diet & Dash Diet Box Set

Negative Calorie Diet & Weight Loss Box Set

Habits of Highly Effective People: What Are the Habits of Successful People?

Slow Cooker: Cookbook with Slow Cooker Recipes

Weight Loss Cookbook: Meal Prep Cookbook for Weight Loss and Clean Eating

Weight Loss Cookbook: Mediterranean Diet for Lasting Weight Loss

Negative Calorie Diet & Dash Diet Box Set

Slow Cooker & Instant Pot Box Set

Children Books: Madison and Astrid's first magical journey & Alice the Superbug Box Set

Belly Diet: The Zero Belly Diet Step-By-Step Guide Which Helps You to Lose Your Belly and Enjoy Your Flat Belly

Weight Loss: 20 Easy and Fast Diet Tips for Losing Weight - An Easy-To-Follow Weight Loss Guide

Instant Pot: Instant Pot Pressure Cooker Cookbook with Easy and Healthy Recipes

Vegan Cookbook: Vegan Cookbook For Beginners, For Kids And For Teens For Diabetics With Pictures

Low Carb: Low Carb Diet Cookbook with Low Carb Keto Recipes for Batch Cooking

Ketogenic Cooking: Ketogenic Cooking With Your Instant Pot

Passive Income: Passive Income Tutorial with 7 Online Ideas to Generate Passive Income Streams for Beginners

Low Carb Diet: Low Carb Diet Recipes Cookbook for Beginners for Batch Cooking

Make Money from Home: How to Make Money Online and Escape the 9-5 Rat Race

Bonus: Subscribe To The Free Weight Loss Report

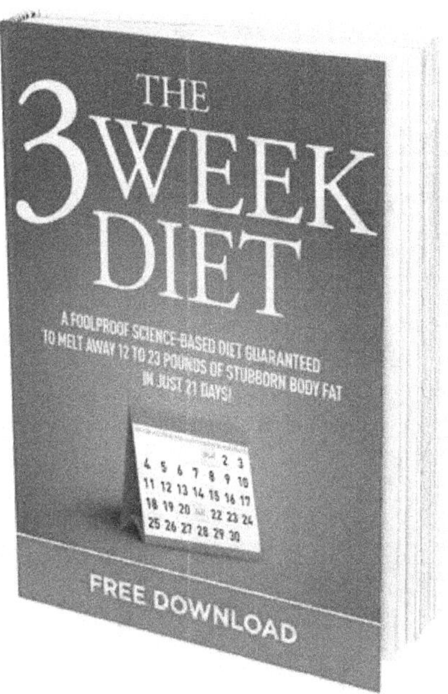

The Introduction Manual is more than just an introduction to the diet. Instead, it discusses the science behind how we gain and lose weight as well as what absolutely needs to be done to attack that stubborn body fat that, until now, has been so challenging to get rid of.

Here are the preview of what you'll get:

- Rapid Weight Loss
- How This System Works
- Why This Diet
- Why 3 Weeks?
- 21 Days To Make A Habit
- Fat Loss VS. Weight Loss
- Nutrients
- Protein, Fat, Carbohydrates
- The Food Pyramid And Obesity
- Fiber
- Metabolism
- How We Get Fat
- Triglycerides
- How To Get Thin
- Diet Overview
- Meal Frequency
- Water
- Diet Essentials
- Let's Get Started

To get instant access to these incredible ebook, go to: http://bit.ly/2tUb9cp